REFLECT TO RESET

YOUR GUIDE TO
MASSIVE
SUCCESS

HALEY SHAW

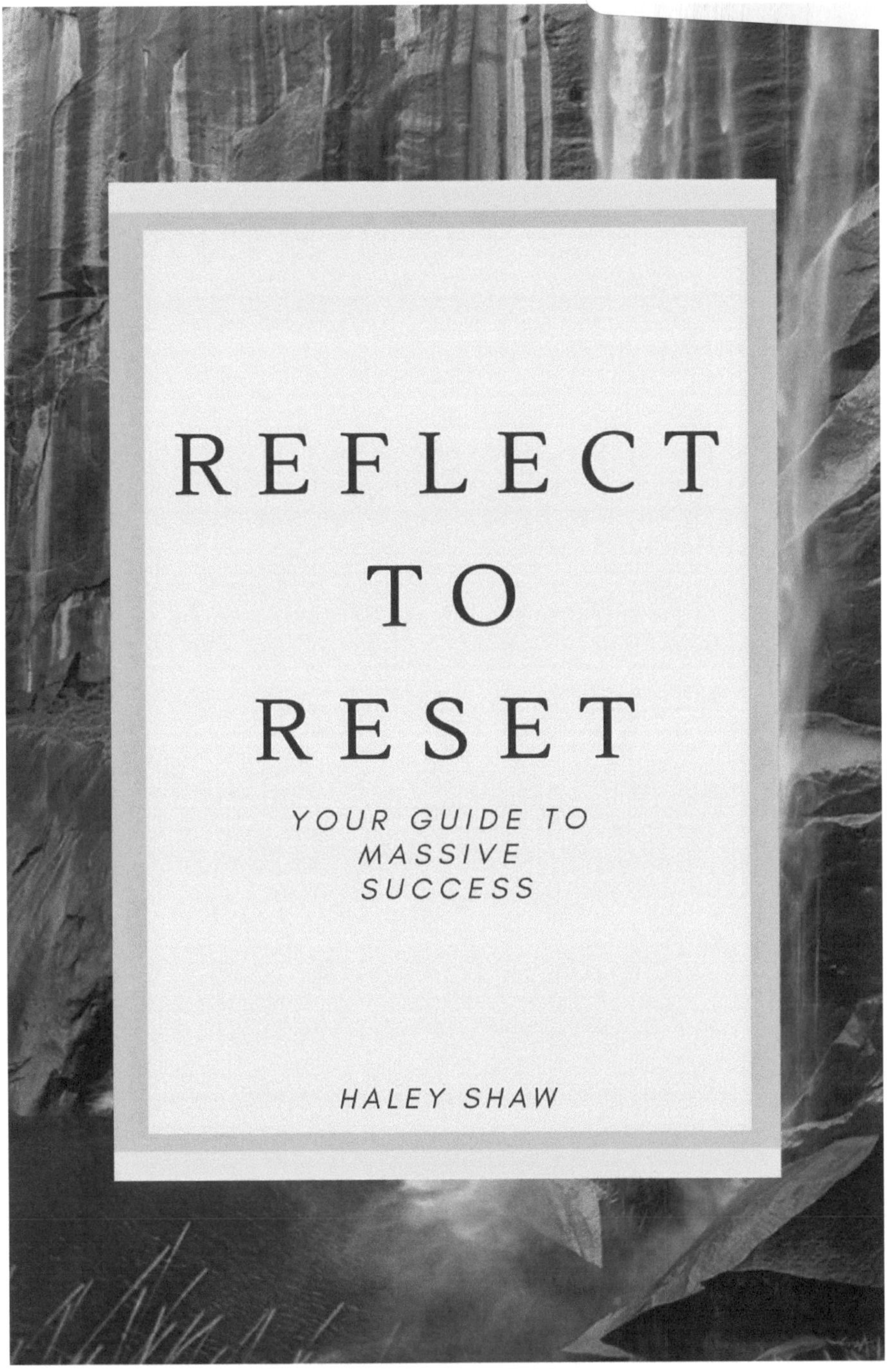

WELCOME MESSAGE: REFLECT TO RESET

Discover your true self & superpower
one day at a time.

While we start the New Year strong, our determination can decrease as life starts to get in the way. You suddenly look up to find the year is well on its way. You're behind on your goals and feeling discouraged. In fact, you feel like you've already failed.

We've all been there and can relate to the impulse to just give up. But if you don't make up the gap this year, it sets you behind when it comes to your goals next year, and the year after that. Settling for 'good enough' today has a cumulative effect on your future and the cost is so much bigger than you can quantify in just six months.

Your Reflect to Reset guide starts with common times of the year individuals look to re-evaluate their goals, and ask themselves:

> *"Are the actions I take today getting me closer to where I want to be?"*

In order to build <u>massive success</u>, we must continually reflect on our past to decide our futures. This can happen any time of year, with most common times listed below.

Times to Reflect:

- Monthly

- Mid-Year as you wrap up second quarter and prepare for the last six months of the year

- After achieving a big goal

- End of year as you prepare your goals for the coming year

Reflection is looking back on the past, **without judgement**, and taking an unbiased inventory of what has happened up to this point. Refrain from assigning good or bad. Just take notice and get a clear picture of how you got here. It is almost like going back in time to take a snapshot of the ingredients of a cake before you made it so you can unpack the parts, better understand the flavor and discover how to adjust it for a different outcome.

Don't give up, get clear on how far you've come and where you want to be. Get started on resetting your year with this guide. You always deserve a **RESET,** and the first step is deciding it (and you) are worth it!

The RESET framework works like this:
Reflect on your past and decide your future

Evaluate your priorities to pursue the right goals

Simplify instead of overcomplicating

Establish a plan to achieve better results in less time

Time Block actions that fast track extraordinary results

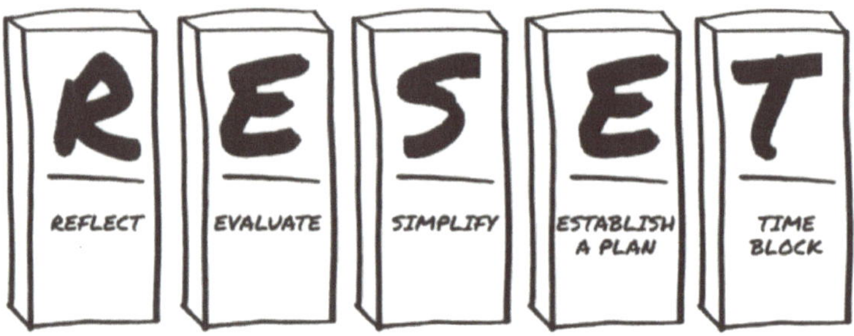

Use this Reflect to Reset guide to build massive success anytime of the year. Take a few minutes daily to ask yourself the questions outlined throughout your guide.

TIPS:

√ Set a 5-minute reminder on your phone
√ Grab a friend, family member, love one, or colleague to support you with these questions
√ Go for a quick walk before or after
√ Listen to happy, up-beat music
√ Devote an area in your home, outside, work, airplane *(perks not having WIFI...sometimes)* or coffee shop for reflection

TABLE OF CONTENTS:

PART I:
REFLECT TO RESET

Discover your true self & superpower
one day at a time.

REFLECT:

YOUR YEAR IN 2 SENTENCES:

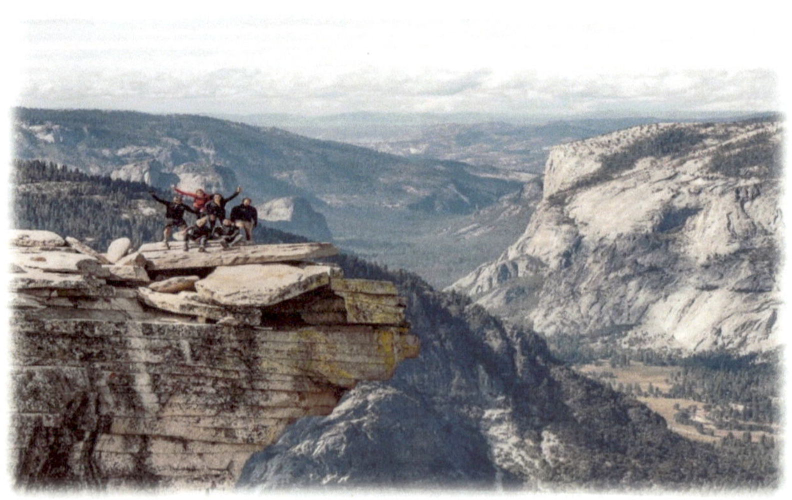

DATE:

REFLECT:

STANDOUTS

- SONGS:

____
____
____
____
____
____
____

- FEELINGS:

____
____
____
____
____
____
____
____

DATE:

REFLECT:

STANDOUTS

- o BOOKS:

- o SOUNDS:

REFLECT:

DATE:

REFLECT:

STANDOUTS

- TRAVEL:

- TASTES:

REFLECT:

DATE:

REFLECT:

STANDOUTS

- SMELLS:

____

____

____

____

____

____

____

- MOVIES/TV:

____

____

____

____

____

____

____

REFLECT:

DATE:

REFLECT → RESET:

List 1-2 of your favorite STANDOUTS from the year below:

STANDOUTS
- o SONGS:

- o FEELINGS:

- o BOOKS:

- o SOUNDS:

- o TRAVEL:

- o TASTES:

- o SMELLS:

- o MOVIES/TV:

RESET:

Now let's evaluate and establish a plan to achieve results.

HOW WILL YOU INCORPORATE THESE STANDOUT MOMENTS MORE IN YOUR LIFE?

WHEN WILL YOU INCORPORATE THESE STANDOUT MOMENTS MORE IN YOUR LIFE?

Breaktime! It is time to color.
Grab some utensils and get to work.

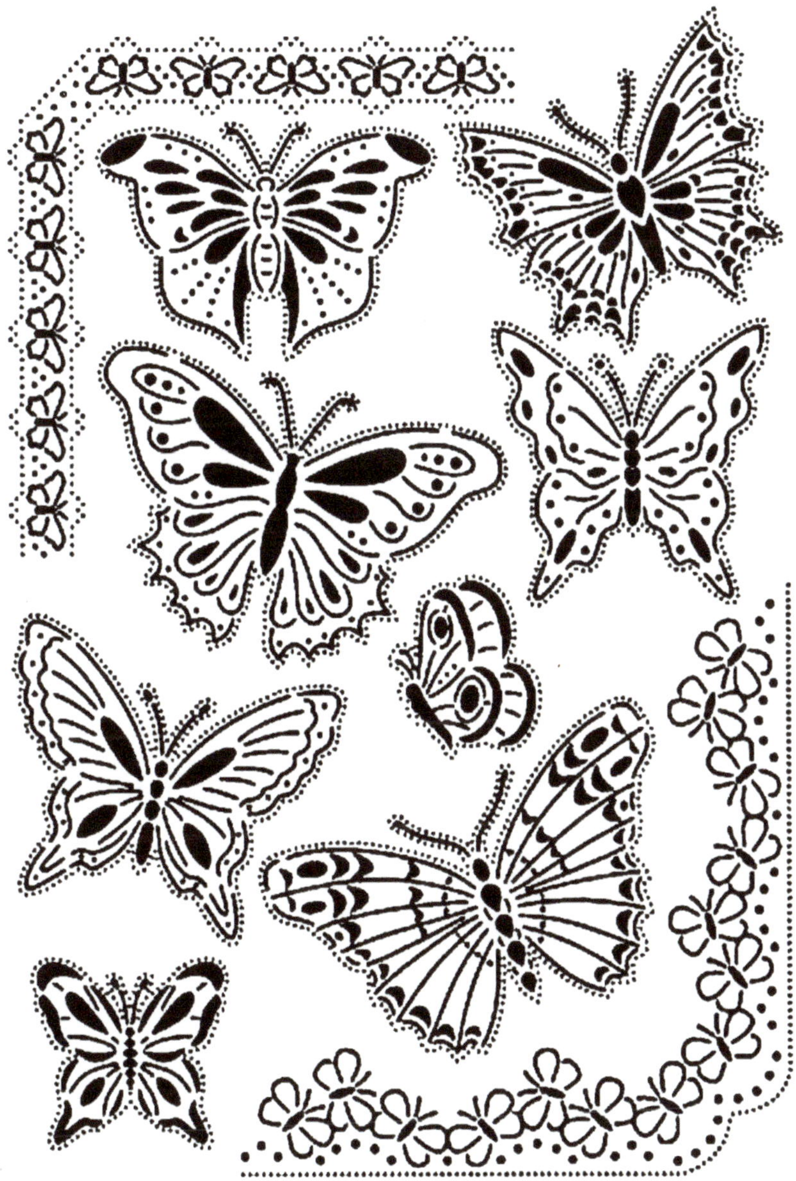

DATE:

REFLECT:

WHAT SURPRISED YOU MOST THIS YEAR?

WHAT WAS THE BEST PART OF YOUR TYPICAL DAY?

DATE:

REFLECT:

WHAT WAS THE GREATEST ADVENTURE(S) THIS YEAR?

WHO WAS THEIR FOR YOU THE MOST THIS YEAR?
NAME ALL THE PEOPLE AND WHY:

DATE:

REFLECT:

WHAT WERE YOUR BIGGEST...

FAILURES:	WINS:
-	-

WHAT DID YOU LEARN?

____

____

____

HOW DID THESE MAKE YOU FEEL?

____

____

____

DATE:

REFLECT:

WHAT MADE YOU FEEL...

ENERGIZED:	DRAINED:
-	-

WHAT DID YOU LEARN?

HOW DID THESE MAKE YOU FEEL?

DATE:

REFLECT:

WHAT BROUGHT YOU...

JOYS:	HEARTACHES:
-	-

WHAT DID YOU LEARN?

HOW DID THESE MAKE YOU FEEL?

DATE:

RESOLVE:

YOUR YEAR IN 2 SENTENCES AGAIN:

Living with Resolved can often be interpreted in duality, as being both/and: I will Resolve to set my own course, and I am Resolved in the lot I've been given.

Spend some time on the ways RESOLVE _**impacted**_ yourself this year... Describe your year **AGAIN** in 2 sentences now that you have reflected on the highs, lows, and everyday moment from this past, or current year...

If you are called to write more keep going...

"Resolve can unify a beginning & determine an ending..."

RESOLVE:

PART II: REFLECT TO RESET

Discover your true self & superpower
one day at a time.

Now, continue to write out your goals and reflect on them throughout the year. Once we self-reflect, we to will resolve to reset.

Ask More "What" Questions Than "Why":
"Why" questions can highlight our limitations and stir up negative emotions, while "what" questions help keep us curious and positive about the future.

Ask More "Am I" Questions:
"Am I" questions embark the curious journey we have in our minds. Here you will open up and truly as yourself what you're doing—in the current state (day-after-day; habit-after-habit) getting you closer to where you saw, or see yourself going?

Continue to define your year with these self-reflect questions.

SELF-REFLECT → RESET

DATE:

SELF-REFLECT TO RESET QUESTIONS:

- Am I using my time wisely? If not, how can I improve?

____

____

____

____

____

____

____

____

SELF-REFLECT TO RESET QUESTIONS:

- Am I taking anything for granted?

- Am I employing a healthy perspective?

- Am I living true to myself?

____

____

____

____

____

____

____

- Am I waking up in the morning ready to take on the day?

____

____

____

____

____

____

____

DATE:

SELF-REFLECT TO RESET QUESTIONS

- Am I thinking negative thoughts before I fall asleep?

- Am I putting enough effort into my relationships?

- Am I taking care of myself physically?

- Am I letting matters that are out of my control stress me out?

- Am I achieving the goals that I've set for myself? If not, how can I achieve those goals?

- Who do I need to connect myself with in order to support me in my goals?

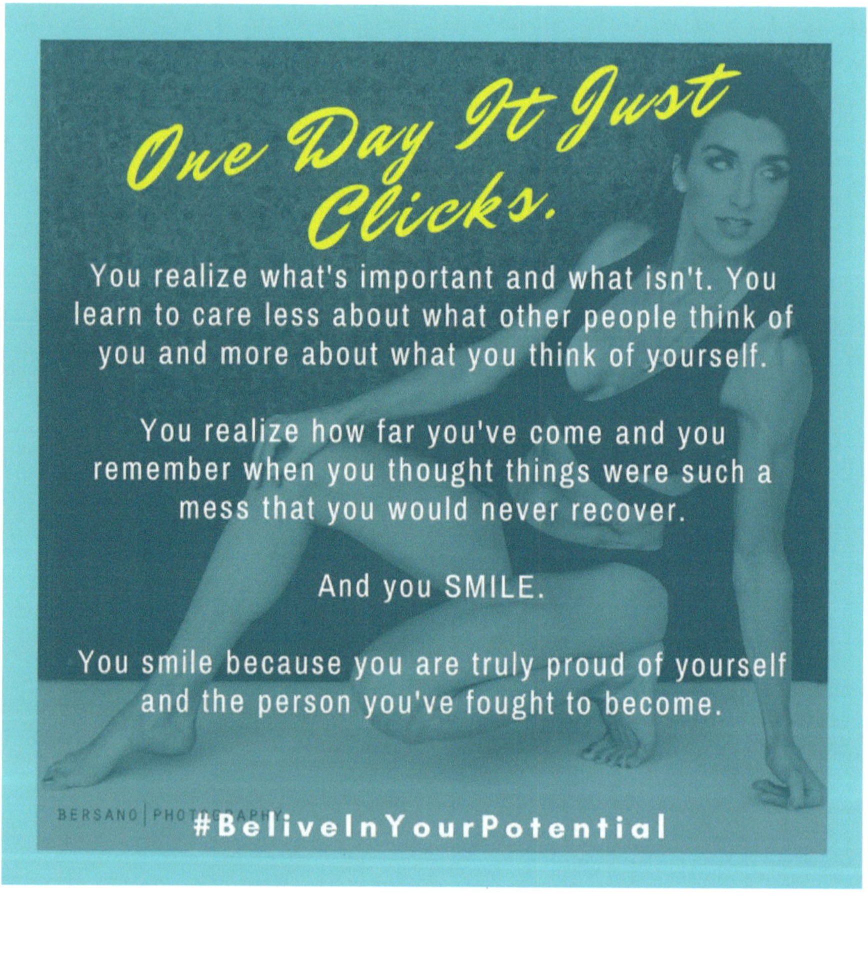

One Day It Just Clicks.

You realize what's important and what isn't. You learn to care less about what other people think of you and more about what you think of yourself.

You realize how far you've come and you remember when you thought things were such a mess that you would never recover.

And you SMILE.

You smile because you are truly proud of yourself and the person you've fought to become.

BERSANO | PHOTOGRAPHY
#BeliveInYourPotential

PART III: REFLECT TO RESET

Discover your true self & superpower
one day at a time.

Top questions to ask yourself every day to get to know yourself better.

- What matters most in my life?

QUESTIONS TO ASK YOURSELF EVERY DAY TO GET TO KNOW YOURSELF BETTER:

STANDOUTS

- What am I doing about the things that matter most in my life?

- If not now, then when?

- When did I last push the boundaries of my comfort zone?

- What small act of kindness was I once shown that I will never forget?

- Is it more important to love or be loved?

- What do I want most in life?

- What is life asking of me?

- Which is worse: failing or never trying?

- If I try to fail and succeed, what have I done?

- What's the one thing I'd like others to remember about me at the end of my life?

- Does it really matter what others think about me?

- To what degree have I actually controlled the course of my life?

- When all is said and done, what will I have said more than I've done?

- Who am I, really?

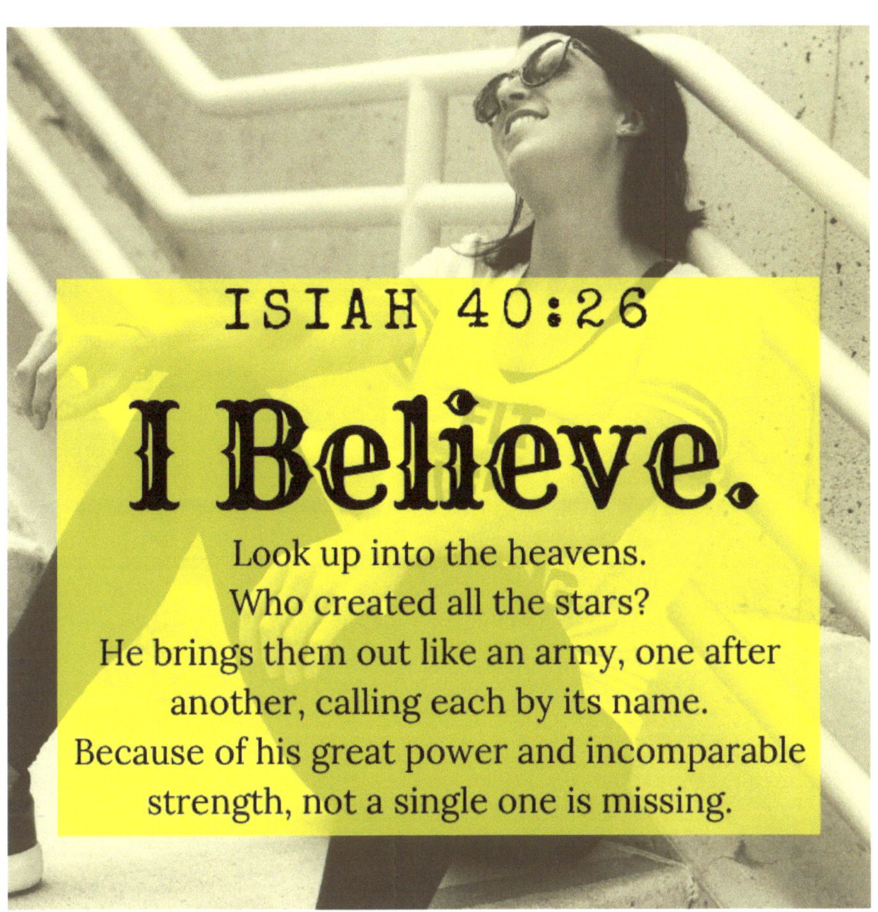

ISIAH 40:26
I Believe.
Look up into the heavens.
Who created all the stars?
He brings them out like an army, one after another, calling each by its name.
Because of his great power and incomparable strength, not a single one is missing.

PART IV:
REFLECT TO RESET

Discover your true self & superpower
one day at a time.

JOURNAL PROMPTS:

WHAT WAS THE BEST PART OF YOUR TYPICAL DAY?

JOURNAL PROMPTS:

WHAT DID YOU DO FOR FUN AS A CHILD?

JOURNAL PROMPTS:

THE WORDS I'D LIKE TO LIVE BY ARE...

I REALLY WISH OTHERS KNEW THIS ABOUT ME...

JOURNAL PROMPTS:

WHAT WAS THE GREATEST ADVENTURES THIS YEAR?

JOURNAL PROMPTS:

I COULDN'T IMAGINE LIVING WITHOUT...

NAME A PASSIONATE WAY YOU'VE SUPPORTED A FRIEND
RECENTLY. THEN WRITE DOWN HOW YOU CAN DO THE SAME
FOR YOURSELF.

WHAT DO YOU LOVE ABOUT YOURSELF?

JOURNAL PROMPTS:

WRITE ABOUT A TIME WHEN YOUR WORK FELT REAL, NECESSARY, AND SATISFLYING TO YOU, WHEHTER THE WORK WAS PAID OR UNPAID, PROFESSIONAL OR DOMESTIC, PHYSICAL OR MENTAL.

JOURNAL PROMPTS:

USING 10 WORDS, DESCRIBE YOURSELF:

1.

2.

3.

4.

5.

6.

7.

8.

9.

10.

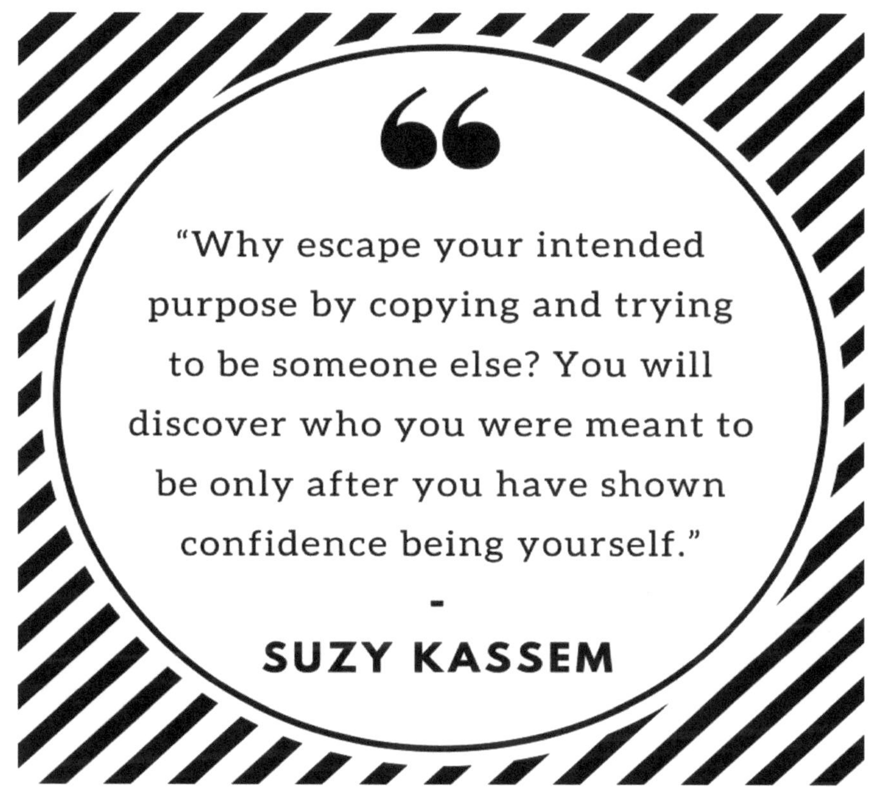

"Why escape your intended purpose by copying and trying to be someone else? You will discover who you were meant to be only after you have shown confidence being yourself."
-
SUZY KASSEM

JOURNAL PROMPTS:

I FEEL MOST ENERGIZED WHEN...

JOURNAL PROMPTS:

WHAT CAN YOU LEARN FROM YOUR BIGGEST MISTAKES?

WHAT CAN YOU LEARN FROM YOUR BIGGEST MISTAKES?

JOURNAL PROMPTS:

WHAT DOES UNCONDITIONAL LOVE LOOK LIKE FOR YOU?

MAKE A LIST OF THE PEOPLE IN YOUR LIFE WHO GENUINELY SUPPORT YOU, AND WHOM YOU CAN GENUINELY TRUST. THEN MAKE TIME TO HANGOUT WITH THEM☺.

PART V: REFLECT TO RESET

Discover your true self & superpower
one day at a time.

CREATE AFFIRMATIONS:

LAST AND SURELY NOT LEAST: CREATING AFFIRNATIONS...

Creating affirmations is a helpful way to clear your mind and put things in perspective. Affirmations can be defined as positives phrases or statements used to challenge negative or unhelpful thoughts. For this exercise, write a list of affirmations in the present tense starting out with the words, "I am…"

For example:

1. I am beautiful, strong, courageous woman.

2. I am a learner at all times and also a teacher.

3. I am a natural born leader.

4. I am pure love and joy.

5. I am child of the Sun. Pure light flows through me and radiates out to bless all beings.

BE BOLD. TAKE RISKS. LIVE LIFE FREELY. LEAD BY EXAMPLE. *TRUST YOUR GUT.* *SAY WHAT YOU FEEL.* **MEAN WHAT YOU SAY.** EXPRESS GRATITUDE. **BELIEVE IN YOUR POWER.** EXCEED YOUR EXPECTATIONS. ***DANCE THE NIGHT AWAY.*** *SKIP DOWN THE STREET.* **DON'T TAKE NO FOR AN ANSWER.** BE YOUR BEST SELF. DON'T LOOK BACK.

XO
Haley Shaw

Thank you for staying true to yourself.

Be proud of who you are.

Never give-up and know the world needs more YOU.

Don't be afraid to leave your mark.

Know your tribe needs you.
Remember I am always here for support.
Work with me to unlock your best YOU!

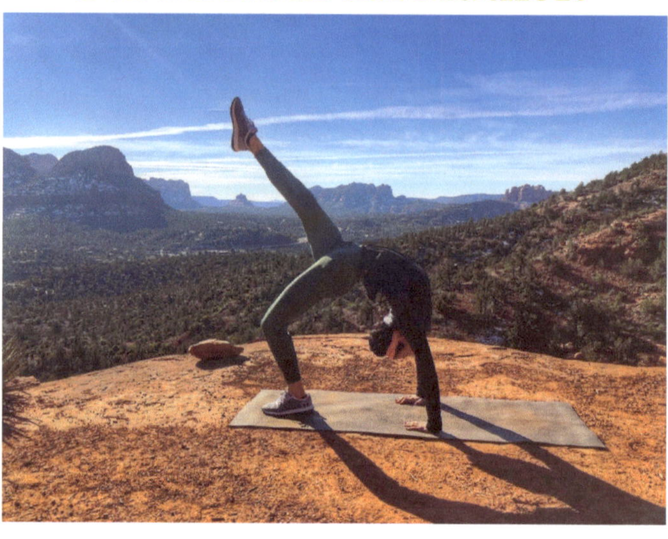

My Personal Mission:
"To help thousands
become confident within themselves
to take on
anything in life!"

About the Author:

Haley Shaw is an Online Health & Fitness Specialist with her company Amp Up Fitness.

Amp Up Fitness specializes in Online Training & Nutrition programs, challenges, and consulting. You can connect with Haley on her website: AmpUpFitness.com where she works with corporations, and individuals nationwide to elevate their health and wellness goals.

Fueled by perseverance; with vivacious, and abundant energy, my skill sets include:

- Looking at life with the glass half FULL, rather than half EMPTY.
- Master Networker, connecting individuals and brands to the ones who need XYZ the most.
- Health Educator & Speaker
- Content Creator for @HaleyAmpUpFit on Instagram and AmpUpFitness.com
- Discover individuals Why through active listening, and consultative selling.
- Community building with innovative ideas
- Group Fitness instructor
- Master Trainer

Social Media Links:

www.AmpUpFitness.com personal website with bio, social links, upcoming events, free resources, online training & nutrition program information

www.LinkedIn.com/in/HaleyAmpUpFit

www.Instagram.com/HaleyAmpUpFit

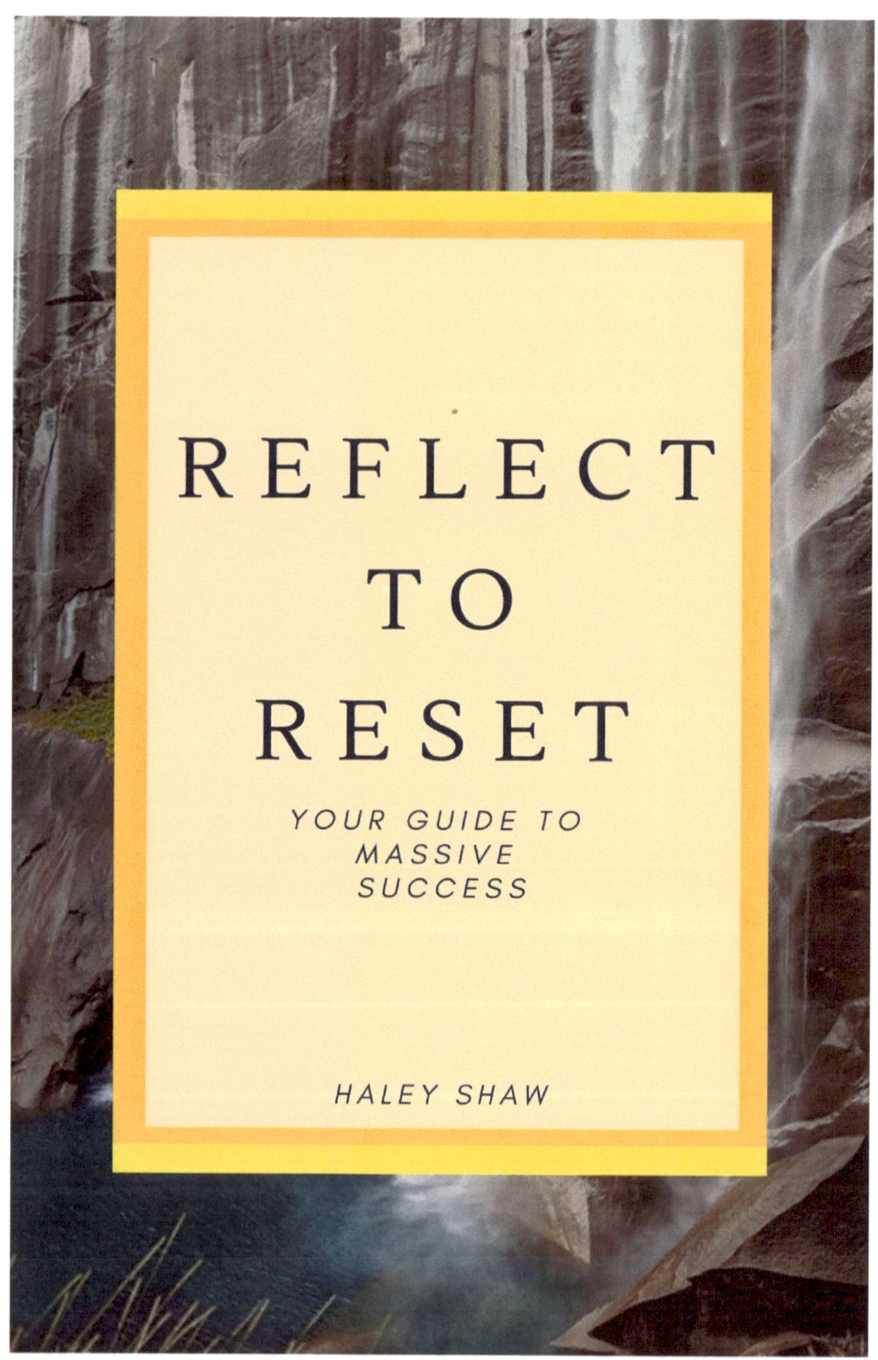
REFLECT
TO
RESET
YOUR GUIDE TO
MASSIVE
SUCCESS
HALEY SHAW

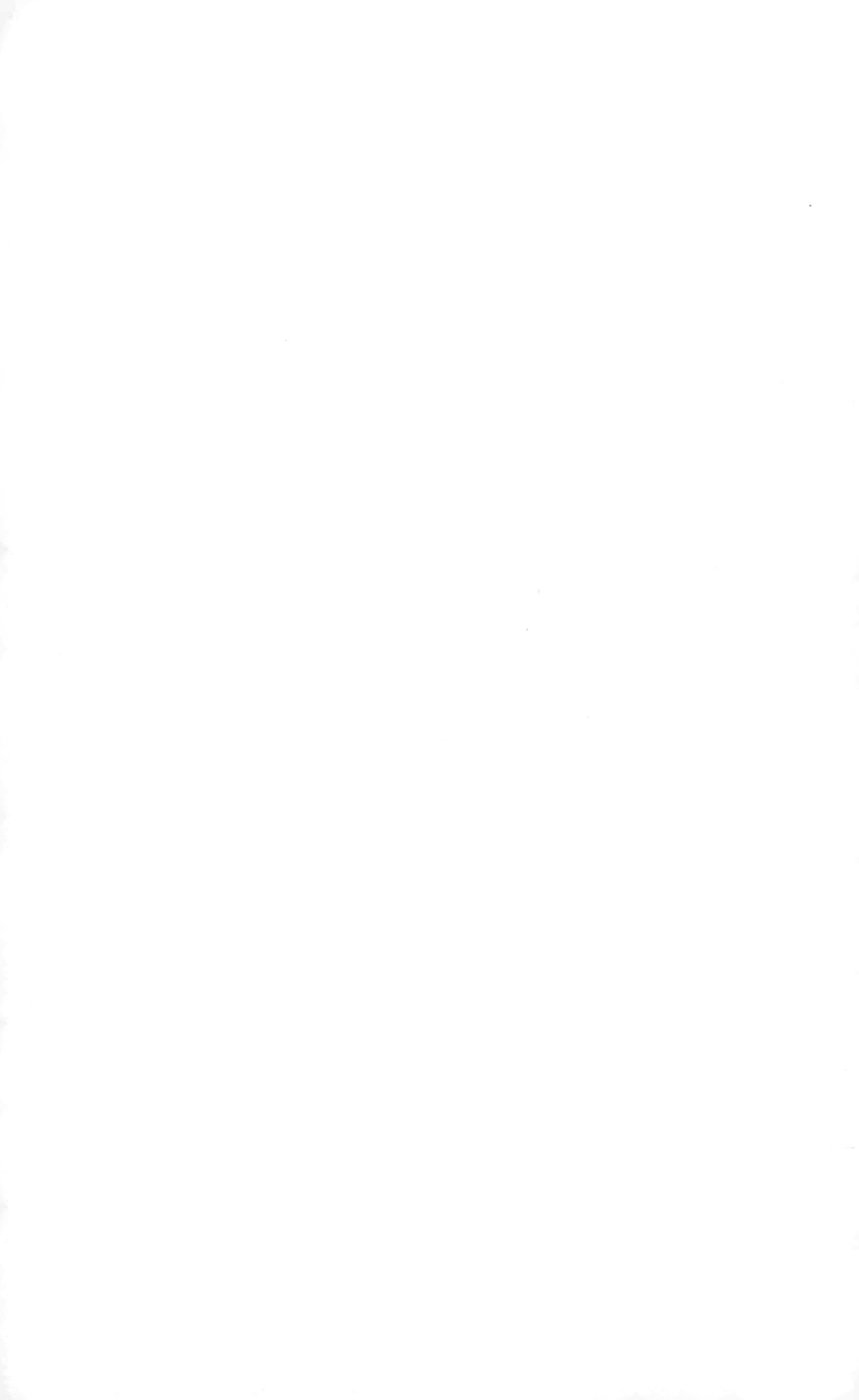